Imagery – The Oldest Form of Healing on the Planet

15 Healing Reasons to Use Your Imagination

Humans have always used their imagination, even before they had a language. Imagery is proven to release natural feel-good chemicals in the body, helping you to manage pain, illness, anger, stress, addiction, sleep, surgery and grief.

In this thought-provoking Itty Bitty® Book, Rhona Jordan identifies 15 reasons to use the power of your mind, among them:

- Heal at home with no down time, side effects, or added expense
- Manage chronic and acute pain
- Reduce or eliminate stress, fear or depression
- Improve brain health

Pick up this book today and learn to use your imagination as a powerful resource for healing.

Your Amazing Itty Bitty® Imagery Book

15 Healing Reasons to Use Your Imagination

Rhona Jordan
C.GIt., C.CHt.

Published by Itty Bitty® Publishing
A subsidiary of S & P Productions, Inc.

Printed in the United States of America

Itty Bitty® Publishing
311 Main Street, Suite D
El Segundo, CA 90245
(310) 640-8885

ISBN: 978-0-9987597-6-0

Photograph of Rhona Jordan courtesy of Prasad Photographer.

This book is dedicated to my husband, John, who silently smiles and observes each new life chapter.

To my gorgeous grandchildren: Jordan, Ryan and Lauren. May your imagination serve your body, mind, and spirit each day of your existence.

To my extraordinary daughter, Heather, who came into this world with pure unconditional love, a teacher and friend to all who know her.

To my wonderful son-in-law, Henry, who constantly encourages me to rise above myself.

For my dear, longtime friend and neighbor, Colleen, who knew exactly how to help me get this book written. Colleen, you imagined enough for both of us.

Stop by our Itty Bitty® website to find interesting blog entries regarding imagery and healing.

www.IttyBittyPublishing.com

Or visit Rhona Jordan at

www.rhonaimagery.com

Table of Contents

Introduction

Heal Yourself Using Imagery

The United States Department of Health and Human Services estimates that more than six million Americans across the country, including such venerable medical facilities as the Mayo Clinic, the Cleveland Clinic and New York City's Columbia University Medical Center, use imagery for healing. The U.S. Department of Veteran's Affairs uses imagery to help veterans recover from Post-Traumatic Stress Disorder. Kaiser Permanente Medical Center, Hoag Hospital and St. Joseph Hospital in California have made imagery CDs available for their patients' use.

In using imagery for healing, Rhona employs the theories of quantum physics, the field of all possibilities. Any time you have a thought, creation begins. If you want to know what your life will be like tomorrow, notice your thoughts/imagination today. Each impulse of experience is metabolized into the molecules of your body. What your mind imagines, your body reflects. In this Itty Bitty® book, you will learn that:

- Your imagination is a constant creator.
- You are the creator, the creation and the observer of your creation.

- Your imagination is powerful beyond measure and this can be applied effectively to healing a range of challenges

This Itty Bitty® book will show you 15 healing reasons for your most powerful built-in resource, your imagination.

Healing Reason 1
Chronic or Acute Pain
Imagery Connects You Deeply to Your Senses and Emotions

Imagery activates your autonomic nervous system. It activates the internal command post deep in the brain that regulates body function. Neuroscientists know that your thoughts are powerful.

1. Chronic pain is ongoing, long-term pain and its treatment is different from acute pain treatment.
2. Acute pain is specific to an immediate, short-term experience; it could result from surgery or a broken bone.
3. The experience of pain can be profoundly affected by the imagination.
4. Using imagery in both chronic and acute pain, the pain can be turned down and you help yourself regain control.
5. What you think becomes your biology by changing the molecular drama within every cell.
6. You are powerful beyond measure; being aware of your body and mind connection effectively reduces chronic and acute pain and accelerates healing.

Examples of Using Imagery in Pain Management

Imagery and Acute Pain:

- A soldier at the front line is seriously injured during battle and hardly notices the pain because the soldier's thoughts (the imagination) are only on survival and going home.
- When a child falls and skins her knee, she asks her mommy to kiss it. Mommy kisses the knee, the pain is gone, and the child happily skips away.

Imagery and Chronic Pain:

- Opiate-based medications over time become less effective and the patient takes more or even a higher dosage, carrying a big risk of dependency, and of course, producing significant side effects.
- People who suffer chronic long-term pain can become dependent on medications and health care providers, eventually feeling overwhelmed with a sense of hopelessness.

You can release your own natural morphine. This is your inner-body pharmacy at work!

Healing Reason 2
Childbirth
Your Body is a Field of Living Information and Intelligence; Through It You Express the Creative Flow of Life

During pregnancy, your body is your baby's universe. A sensation, pleasurable or uncomfortable, imaginary or real, changes your body and the body of your unborn baby on a cellular, molecular level. Your thoughts, your imagination, are literally made into flesh.

1. Your thoughts, feelings, and environment, all affect your baby.
2. When you are nurturing yourself and avoiding toxic situations, your body is in balance and so is your unborn baby.
3. When you are calm, your baby is calm.
4. Adrenaline, noradrenaline, oxytocin and serotonin are messenger molecules traveling across the placenta, and those powerful chemicals influence your baby.

The Role of Imagery for You and Baby

- Studies using ultrasound monitoring clearly showed that within moments after a pregnant woman experienced a stressful event, her unborn baby responded with an accelerated heart rate.
- Your little one is adaptable, resilient, aware and responsive to you.

You Can Use Imagery to Prepare for the Birth.

- Mentally travel inside the universe of your body and pass through the uterine wall honoring this lifeline that is feeding and nourishing your baby.
- Talk to your baby and say that soon you will be holding the little one in your arms.
- Imagine an easy, comfortable birth.
- Imagine your body in the most relaxed state, loving and happy.
- Remind yourself that the body is filled with intelligence and information and it knows exactly what to do.

Healing Reason 3
Cancer Cells and Chemotherapy
are Energy

Every cell in your body is filled with intelligence and knows on a chemical level your every thought, word, action and re-action for healing.

1. Imagery encourages healthy cells to reproduce.
2. Your thoughts and imagination focused on healing are more powerful than any cancer cell.
3. Frequency and vibration is the "you" vibrating in the quantum field; the field where all possibility and creations manifest to heal.
4. When chemo is imagined as healing energy, there are fewer side effects.

Imagery is Completely Compatible with Chemotherapy

- When experiencing chemotherapy, imagine it as liquid light or energy that is moving the molecules and cells.
- When you imagine chemo viewed as poison, the body reacts accordingly and may experience many side effects.
- Imagine and talk directly to the cancer cells.
- Give the cancer cells permission to leave the body.
- Imagine talking to millions of healthy cells, reminding them they are powerful beyond measure.
- Imagine billions more healthy cells flowing from every direction into existence.

Healing Reason 4
Stress, Fear or Depression
Imagery Creates a Safe Place for the Mind

The body reflects every emotional feeling and reacts the same, whether the emotion is from a real or imagined event; either one can create stress, fear or depression.

1. Stress, fear or depression affect the autoimmune system, nervous system, heart rate, blood pressure, breathing rhythm, elimination, digestion, sleep and energy levels.
2. Because these emotions affect us on a cellular level, they negatively influence our immune system's healing abilities.
3. These powerful emotions take our thinking offline, creating confusion and memory loss.
4. None of us can make accurate or clear decisions when we are upset.

Your Imagination is the Most Important and Valuable Natural Resource You Have

- Change is constant in life and it is the unknown that makes life an adventure.
- Invite yourself to be comfortable with the unknown and with change.
- How you deal with fear is important because it affects you on a cellular level and influences your immune system's healing abilities.
- Serotonin is a natural chemical the body creates, lifting your spirits up by producing a natural high.
- Imagine your body producing serotonin and the messenger molecules allowing the body to feel stress-less, safe and happy.

"Imagination is more important than knowledge."
-- Albert Einstein

Healing Reason 5
Preparing for Surgery – Imagine that Hands of Light are Touching You

When we are facing a surgical procedure that is voluntary, perhaps for a firmer chin or straighter nose, we get excited for the new look and hardly think about the surgical procedure. However, when we are facing a surgery because of a dysfunction, such as organ failure or the result of a serious illness, the feelings can be fear, hopelessness or dread, and are intensified, thus compromising the immune system.

1. It is very important to speak to the organ or body part that is leaving the body.
2. Thank it for being with you and serving you well all these years.
3. Tell it that soon it will be released for the good of the whole body, and with gratitude, once again thank it, and say it will be missed and is loved. "Good bye."
4. This information prepares and alerts the chemistry, cells, molecules, blood flow, tissues, organs, bones and all systems for the procedure.

Preparing for the Actual Surgery

Bearing in mind that using your imagination, you are powerful beyond measure:

- Give yourself permission to sleep peacefully the night before the procedure.
- On the day of the surgery, know that the room is being prepared for you.
- The smiling staff is waiting for your arrival and each well-trained, educated doctor, nurse and aid are all energy healers with hands of light; smile with them.
- Imagine directing your blood pressure to remain normal, with little need for bleeding, while the body sleeps gently, deeply, safely and comfortably during the entire procedure.
- When the IV is attached, look up at the bag of fluids and imagine that liquid as light or energy supporting your well-being.
- Smile with gratitude as the liquid light joins the fluid tides within your body.
- After the procedure, you awaken, comfortable and surprised it is over, smiling, resting and healing.
- Imagine talking to the incision area and telling the body it is safe and can heal easily, perfectly and quickly.

Healing Reason 6
Healing Grief

Energy always changes form, it never stays the same. Like boiling water turns into steam, then turns into vapor, you can't see it, but is it there; it is energy changing form. Grief never leaves us where it found us. Grief can occur over the loss of a pet, a family member, a job, a marriage, even an irreplaceable photo or special piece of jewelry. Grief is a form of energy.

1. When deep, inconsolable feelings of sadness are overwhelming, so are the physical reactions in our body.
2. We can even die from grief, as in 2017, when Debbie Reynolds, grieving over the death of her daughter, Carrie Fisher, died within two days of her daughter.
3. Holidays and special anniversaries related to grief are often played out in our body by developing a common cold or some other illness, or feeling the need for isolation.
4. Many people experience depression around calendar events, even though they don't consciously remember it as a calendar event.
5. Death or loss requires closure and ways to manage our emotions.

Dealing with Grief

Time helps, but time is not the healer. Here is an example of the use of imagination to heal a sense of loss:

I imagined that my friend, Fran, was in the front passenger seat and as I drove and talked to her, would even tell her to buckle her seat belt for the ride to the store. The images were so strong that I imagined I could hear her laugh at the daily stories, and at the same time, my physical body was releasing cortisol and creating serotonin. Imagining with Fran got me through the first few years of my close friend's death.

- Your imagination is available to you all the time for closure; to share joy or sorrow, or anything else that was left unsaid.
- Your imagination supports your healing through the grief journey that never leaves you where it found you.

Healing Reason 7
Addiction
You are Stronger

The brain is precious and important because it controls everything in your body; words you say, the choices you make, who you marry, where you work, what you wear, who you love – the list is endless. With imagery, it is possible to surround yourself with the healthy brain's natural high that is real, beautiful and profound. Maintaining a healthy brain is the smartest decision you can ever make.

1. Experimenting with chemicals to alter the brain chemistry has a **NO WIN** ending.
2. Destructive daily addictions to video games or your own cellphone keeps you isolated from others.
3. Some people are addicted to sweets and hide them around the house in the same way an alcoholic hides the bottles.
4. Whatever the addiction, it is polarity or extremes that keep you out of balance with yourself, the world, and everyone in it.

Live Free of Addiction

Every year, from birthday to birthday, we travel around the Sun. This year, pack lighter and leave the addictions behind. Enjoy your brain and the journey. Cheers! You are a world traveler. Imagine that!

- When you find yourself losing control with choices that do not serve you, imagine yourself saying NO to yourself.
- Turn around and walk away.
- You are now stepping back into your power and re-creating you as the person with a healthy, balanced brain instead of the Scarecrow in the Wizard of Oz, who always wanted a brain.

Healing Reason 8
Sleep
Begin and End Each Day in Gratitude

Therapeutic sleep for seven or eight hours encourages the body to regenerate and heal. Sometimes we fall asleep, but can't seem to stay asleep longer than 4 or 5 hours. When we don't get enough sleep, we are tired and cranky. According to Chinese medicine, each organ needs time to repair during sleep and if we wake up too soon, that process is not complete.

1. Melatonin is the body's natural chemical that is released for sleep.
2. Cortisol is the body's natural chemical released during stress.
3. Sleep is a state of consciousness.
4. Dreaming is a state of consciousness.
5. You can use your imagination to attain better sleep!

Use your Imagination for Better Sleep

- Consider imagining the body is turning down the cortisol and turning up and releasing more melatonin supporting your sleep until the appropriate hour to awaken.
- Make it as real as you can, talk to your body, too.
- Imagine that the list of all the things that you have to do or are concerned about is sitting across the room on the shelf and tomorrow you can pick it up again, but for tonight, for right now, you want to sleep.
- Imagine you are giving yourself permission to rest your body and sleep comfortably.
- Feel the blanket, the safety of the room, and your eyelids closing down from all the activity of the day as droplets of melatonin signal the response to relax your shoulders and back and legs.
- Yawn and stretch as the breathing slows down and you comfortably settle in for the night.
- One by one, name what you are grateful for as your body begins to slumber.

Healing Reason 9
Chronic Anger

When anger is experienced every day, not just on occasion, it can kill you.

1. Observing your anger triggers is a big step in learning to manage your emotions and react differently.
2. Anger is related to: heart disease, diabetes, smoking, depression, drug use, disassociation with family and friends, isolation, blaming others, and weight gain (potentially consuming an extra 600 calories daily).
3. Anger can kill you by producing high levels of stress hormones, thus speeding the buildup of plaque in the arteries.

Antidotes to Anger

Gratitude changes the chemistry in the body by turning down the stress hormones, cortisol and adrenaline. When you are in gratitude, your body chemistry releases a healing combination of serotonin, endorphins, dopamine, and oxytocin. These feel-good chemicals enhance our immune system, encourage clear thinking, and manage gut reactions.

- Replace anger with gratitude.
- Imagine making a conscious choice to become supportive of your wellbeing.

Know that your emotional words change the biology of those you are speaking to. Your anger affects everyone you are in contact with. When you say to someone, "I don't like you," that person's immune system is compromised and they feel awful, too.

- Become aware of the emotional words you use.
- Every action and every reaction … is a choice.

Healing Reason 10
Trichotillomania (Trich) – Body-Focused Repetitive Behaviors

Trichotillomania is stimulation or over self-stimulation behavior exhibited by people of all ages, from babies to adults.

1. We do not yet know why this behavior occurs.
2. Trich behaviors include chronic cheek biting, hair-pulling, nail-biting, and picking the skin around nail beds or different parts of the body.
3. These behaviors can occur on a person's own body or that of a pet or doll.
4. Many people pick or pull when watching television or sitting in a car, feeling tired, bored, fussy, falling asleep or when waking up.
5. Trich is being researched and behavioral tools and some medications are helping.
6. Saying "Stop, don't pull or pick!" is not always the most effective deterrent.

Ways to Deal with Nail-Biting, Skin-Picking or Hair-Pulling

Use your imagination to focus the body and mind in a new direction and develop successful strategies for dealing with Trich struggles:

- Decide to overcome a repetitive behavior that does not serve you.
- Feel good about your decision to not bite, pick or pull.
- Be consciously aware of when and where the body-focused behavior may be triggered and prepare for those times with tools and self-talk.
- Picture your nails as healthy and beautiful.
- Tell your hair it is where it needs to grow, and that is not on the floor.
- Use tools to disrupt the repetitive pattern.
- Reach for a tool to feel a different stimulation.
- Use a doll instead of your own hair.
- Offer a rattle, touch toys, fiddle toys, a ball that can be squeezed, or a special feeling blanket to a small baby.
- Wear gloves at night.

Healing Reason 11
The Importance of Brain Health

Every decision you make, from your financial income to who you marry, is dictated by the health of your brain.

1. Inside the skull are many sharp edges covering the brain.
2. When the skull is hit hard enough for the brain to slosh around, it can bruise, bleed, or swell; it is injured.
3. An injury may not show up at the time of the incident, but many years later, your behavior can be affected.
4. A damaged brain can change your life and every decision you make and can cause dementia, paranoia, suicidal thoughts, attention deficit disorder, conduct disorder; create rage, chronic anger, seizures – the list is endless.
5. Football players are constantly being hit, but the damage may not show up until much later in life.
6. Soccer players think it is fun to bounce a soccer ball off their heads; in that one second, life as you know it can change forever.

How to Care for Your Brain

The importance of healthy brain education begins with all parents, teachers, sports coaches, and most importantly, with ourselves.

- Take as good care of your brain as you would a newborn baby.
- Your brain serves you from your first breath to your last.
- Treat your brain with enormous respect.
- Imagine you are making the right decision to maintain a healthy brain.
- Imagine the right choices you are making because of a healthy brain.
- Imagine protecting the brains of your children.
- Imagine saying "NO!" to danger and "YES!" to a healthy brain.

Healing Reason 12
Quantum Physics and the Body

You are stardust, atoms, molecules, earth minerals and consciousness. You are powerful beyond measure.

1. Every atom in your body has the same components of a collapsed star; in this sense, you are the star you have been wishing upon and your body is made from stardust.
2. Magnesium, iron and salt are minerals found in your body and in the earth.
3. You are made of the same stuff as the galaxies and the earth.
4. You may think that your body and the chair you are sitting on are solid; both are billions of molecules spinning in space.
5. When you grasp that thought, creation begins; you are co-creator with the universe.
6. Your heart sends out electromagnetic energy that pulls you to wonderful people, events and opportunities.
7. Quantum physicists say that when their equipment is developed, the magnetic measurement from the heart will reach infinity.

What Will You Manifest for Yourself?

Today the body is printing out the thoughts you had yesterday. When you understand the mechanics of quantum physics and working with consciousness, you become profoundly aware how the energies of your thoughts and words are created and become your reality.

- Imagine what you want to create: spiritually, health, wealth, relationships?
- Imagine your thoughts and words as the particle, or the wave, of creation pulled to you.

Healing Reason 13
Conscious Eating
Spiritual and Body Awareness

You are a spiritual being in an earth body suited
to this galaxy. The food you eat becomes part of
your skin-encapsulated ego. Eating consciously is
very different from just chomping food down and
running to start the next project.

1. All food is energy, frequency, and
    vibration and this varies by the colors of
    the food.
2. While you are eating, if your mind is
    elsewhere, you aren't able to really enjoy
    the many different tastes, colors, textures,
    and smells of the delicious food.
3. Eating consciously precludes all other
    distractions such as watching television
    or working at your desk.
4. Eating consciously means looking at
    what is on the plate, appreciating it and
    how the synchronicity of events landed it
    on the plate; where it came from, how it
    was grown or produced, how well it was
    prepared.

You Are What You Eat!

Being consciously aware of the food changes it on a molecular level as it enters your body. This supports your body's powerful healing immune system and lines your stomach with new cells every three days.

- Purchase or choose foods of many different colors to eat.
- While preparing the food, bless it and infuse the meal with love.
- While eating consciously, notice the color, fragrance, texture and temperature of the food.
- Savor the food while chewing slowly as all the flavors are released and the gut is better able to digest it.
- Imagine the food as light or energy entering your body.
- Imagine the strength the food gives to your bones, muscles, cells and molecules.
- Eating in this way, you will feel fuller sooner, supporting your ideal weight and general good health.

Healing Reason 14
Interstitial Cystitis
Inflammation of the Bladder and its Lining, Urinary Symptoms, Pain, and Pelvic Floor Dysfunction

For people with interstitial cystitis, every day presents new challenges. Most of the women and some of the men I work with at the clinics share these experiences and fears:

1. Finding public bathrooms.
2. Handling the stress of this condition.
3. Canceling a much-needed vacation.
4. Flare-ups; the pain getting worse.
5. Eliminating foods/drinks because of pain.
6. Painful sex; tail bone, belly or inner thigh pain.
7. Fear of bladder never healing.
8. Unending doctor visits, medical tests, prescriptions and procedures.
9. Feeling alone and/or overwhelmed.
10. Experiencing referred pain in a different part of the body than the actual site of the pain stimulus; like a heart attack felt in the neck and back rather than the chest.
11. Tight pelvic floor muscles that irritate nerves, causing triggers that affect other organs.

You Can Take Control to Get Your Life Back

With holistic, multiple approaches, combinations of treatments, therapies and diet alterations, it is a long journey, but you can get your life back. Stretching, exercising and moving the body is essential. Imagery can be very effective during your journey. Here is a relaxing bath technique to lessen symptoms and promote healing.

- Stretch the body, taking a few deep breaths; give your body permission to heal itself; tell it that you love yourself unconditionally right now.
- Light a candle and set the mood, then step into a warm bath.
- Feel the warm waters relaxing the pelvic floor muscles that hold the bladder in place; imagine the bladder floating.
- Imagine the nerve endings calming down, cooling the urethra, bladder and its lining as they are healing.
- As the nervous system calms down, bladder urgency is less and less and less.
- Talk to your listening body, it wants to be well.
- Imagine having your life back and make it as real as you can in your mind.
- When you empty the bathtub, imagine the discomfort being washed away.
- Let go of the outcome and experience, being fully in the moment.

Healing Reason 15
Meditation

Meditation is a tool that can be used for managing and discovering the body's intelligence.

1. It has been used for thousands of years and serious modern scientists started studying it around 1970.
2. Because of the science behind meditation, scientists are attending meditation retreats to improve their cognitive and emotional skills.
3. Meditation not only changes brain neuronal interconnections, but also increases brain tissue volume, increases telomerase activity which lengthens your lifespan, and diminishes inflammation and other biological stresses that occur at the molecular level.
4. Meditation is silent intelligence, the single, most powerfully direct means to connect with the mind's deeper level, activating a hidden force.
5. Meditation supports stronger physical and emotional health.
6. Two thirty-minute meditations in the same day give your body the rest of a full night's sleep.

Benefits of Daily Meditation

- Reduces stress and over-reaction.
- Opens creativity and the desire to create.
- Supports better decision making.
- Improves executive functions.
- Increases learning ability.
- Increases levels of intelligence.
- Calms and balances mind and spirit.
- Improves immune system function.
- Enhances healthy growth of brain matter.
- Expands awareness with right actions.

Beyond the practice of daily meditation by individuals, consider the following:

- Imagine students in every classroom meditating together.
- Imagine families meditating together.
- Imagine the Armed Forces meditating together.
- Imagine the government meditating together.

You've Finished. Before You Go…

Tweet/share that you finished this book.

Please star rate this book.

Reviews are solid gold to writers. Please take a few minutes to give us some itty bitty feedback.

ABOUT THE AUTHOR

Rhona first experienced Guided Imagery and Clinical Hypnosis when she was scheduled for a serious cancer surgery. The imagery was powerful and Rhona breezed through the procedure and recovered ahead of schedule. This life-changing event motivated Rhona to learn more about these powerful techniques.

An avid believer in the power of imagery, Rhona stays on the cutting edge. Her academic background spans the study of Regression Therapy in New Delhi, India, to her recent graduation from Chopra University, where she qualified as a global Primordial Sound Meditation instructor for the Chopra Center for Wellbeing.

Rhona currently works from four clinics in Orange County, California, offering imagery and hypnosis to patients during their medical procedures, and maintains her private practice in Orange. She also offers free monthly meditations at a local hospital in Newport Beach.

Awarded Humanitarian of the Year by the Trauma Intervention Program for her work with trauma victims and first responders, Rhona is a sought-after motivational speaker. You can reach her at her website: www.rhonaimagery.com or by email at: Rhonaimagery@aol.com

Imagine what can be achieved!

If you enjoyed this Itty Bitty® Book you might also enjoy or benefit from:

- **Your Amazing Itty Bitty® Cancer Book** – Jacqueline Kreple

- **Your Amazing Itty Bitty® Self-Hypnosis Book** – Amy Mayne Robinson, CHt

- **Your Amazing Itty Bitty® Affirmations Book** – Micaela Passiri

And many other Itty Bitty® books available online.

Made in the USA
San Bernardino, CA
18 June 2017